How to Help Your Doctor Help *you*

A Patient/Patient Advocate's Guide to Better Healthcare

Dr. Dustie Johnson, PhD

innovativeink
PUBLISHING
A Division of Kendall Hunt

Cover image Shutterstock.com

innovativeink PUBLISHING
A Division of Kendall Hunt

www.innovativeinkpublishing.com
Send all inquiries to:
4050 Westmark Drive
Dubuque, IA 52004-1840

Print ISBN: 979-8-3197-0961-5
eBook ISBN: 979-8-3197-0962-2

Published in the United States of America

Dedication

I would like to dedicate this guide to all the people in my life who have loved, supported, and encouraged me to follow my heart and told me anything is possible. Each one of you have played a part in inspiring the creation of this guide book.

To my Lord and Savior, ***Jesus Christ****, I give all the praise and glory. Thank you for all the blessings in my life and allowing me the opportunity to share this information.*

To my husband **Guy "Jamie" Johnson** *and my son* **Hayden Johnson***, thank you for loving me and supporting everything I do.*

To my **Daddy, Doyle Thompson***, this is a tribute, in loving memory to the man who made me who I am today and never told me I couldn't do anything.*

To my true family and dear friends, you know who each of you are, thank you for loving me and supporting me when the ones who should didn't.

I want to express my gratitude to all of the medical professionals who have cared for me, my family members and dear friends, and those who have encouraged me to finish this so they can share it with their patients.

Contents

Introduction

DISCLAIMER: THE INFORMATION CONTAINED IN THIS GUIDE BOOK IS NOT INTENDED TO PROVIDE ANY MEDICAL ADVICE.

Please let me start by explaining that I am not a medical doctor; I am a scientist with a PhD in reproductive physiology. I am writing this guide as a long-time patient advocate for family and friends and as a patient myself, with the extra benefit of knowledge that my education and work have afforded me. Over the many years of experience with the healthcare system, I have made numerous observations and gathered a great deal of information that God has called on my heart to share.

I have watched as our healthcare system changed from a family physician who knew their patients on a personal level to a much larger, resource- and time-deficient system where there is little personal knowledge of the patients. This does not mean that the physicians and staff are not good at their jobs or do not care, but rather that they do not have the luxury of time to get to know their patients and are limited by the information they have available to them to help you with your care. As such, the burden falls more on the patients themselves and their advocates to help the doctors provide you with the best care. I have written this book so you know what you can do to **Help Your Doctor Help You.**

In this book, I hope to share some information that I have found helpful and that I hope can help you in obtaining the best health care. I will also share some anecdotes along the way on why I found this information so important. These are stories from my own experiences or those of people I know. Names have been left out or changed to protect the privacy of all involved.

1

Be an Active Participant in Your Own Health Care

One of the first things you can do to help make sure you receive better health care is commit to being an active participant in your own health care. This means you need to become knowledgeable about all the things that affect your health and the care you receive. Take charge! Be empowered! Do not be afraid! While I understand that this can seem like an overwhelming task, you have made a great start by picking up this book. While no guide can cover every aspect of your health care, I will try to give you as many tools as I can to help you. I will also show you how to put this information together to make it easier for both you and your health care providers. Let's start with some of the things that you need to know.

Medications

It is very important to know all of the medicines you take and why you take them. This includes any supplements, such as vitamins, dietary aids such as probiotics, or natural remedies such as herbs, and hormone replacements. Yes, this also includes botox injections, weight loss medications, eye drops, nose sprays, and illicit or recreational substances such as marijuana or mushrooms. Many of these substances can interact with medications, cause serious adverse reactions, or make medications ineffective. It is important to make a list of all these

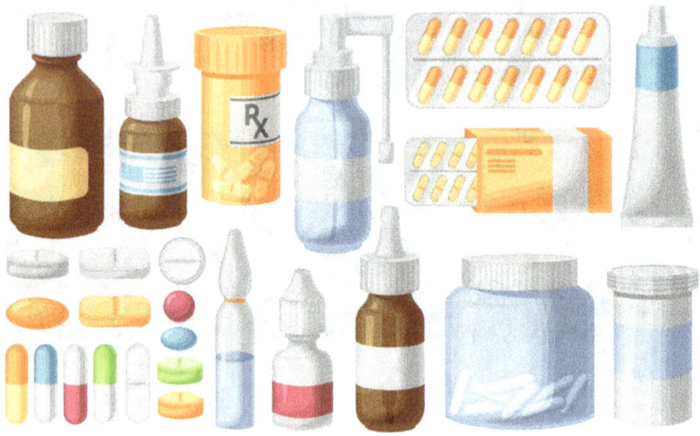
WinWin artlab/Shutterstock.com

medications and supplements along with the doses and instructions (e.g., take one pill twice a day) and why you take them. If you are not sure why you are taking them, be sure to ask your health care provider. Be careful that the spelling is correct. There are many medications that sound very similar but have very different functions.

If your doctor is prescribing a new medication, be sure to ask what it is for, how you are supposed to take it, what side effects you might experience, and whether there are any dangerous symptoms you should be on the lookout for in case you have an allergic reaction.

If you are a patient advocate (we will talk about advocates more in a bit), be sure to know all the patient's medications just as you would for yourself. In fact, you might even want to take a picture of the medication so you can recognize them if they are out of the original prescription bottle, such as in a pill box.

Follow Directions

Part of being an active participant in your care is to take your medicines as they are prescribed. It is also important to take all of the medications your doctor prescribes just as they have ordered. For example, if your doctor has prescribed an antibiotic for an infection, you need to take all of it. If you stop taking it when you start feeling better and do not finish the entire dose, the infection may not be completely cleared up. This can also make the infection become resistant to the antibiotics, meaning that they may not work in the future. Another example is if you are taking blood pressure medicine, you have to take it as prescribed to control your condition all the time, not just when you feel bad.

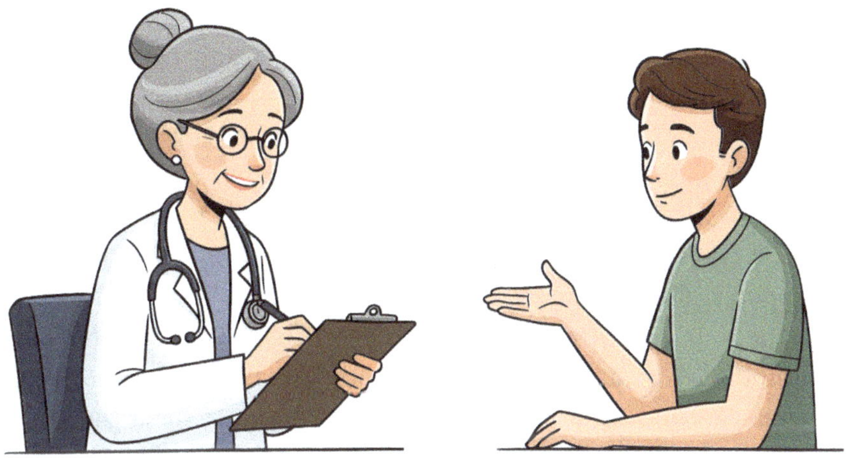

Shahid_Irfan/Shutterstock.com

Communication

Communication is important in all areas of your life, but it is absolutely critical when talking about your health care. It is important to talk to your doctor about your concerns and your healthcare goals and to ask questions. Let me say this again: "ask questions"! Never be afraid to speak up and ask questions, especially if you do not understand what they are telling you. There are never any bad questions. This means you should even ask questions that may seem embarrassing, for instance about your sexual health. Your health care provider should encourage you to share your concerns and be willing to listen. Find a provider that you are comfortable with and who will be a partner in achieving your healthcare goals. **Never settle!** You should choose a healthcare provider that takes the time and treats you with respect. Also remember that it is always OK to ask for a second opinion.

Truth or Consequences

This may sound like a strange title for a section on health care, but it is absolutely critical to receiving the best health care. A healthcare provider may ask you some questions, on their questionnaires or during your visits, that may make you a little uncomfortable. They are not asking these questions to be nosey or to make you squirm; these questions are critical to obtaining all the information they need to help you. Some of these questions may be about your alcohol consumption, smoking or vaping, recreational drug use, or your sexual practices. It is important that you answer these questions fully and truthfully. This can mean the difference between you receiving the proper care and suffering the consequences such as having a bad reaction or missing an important condition that will be fine if treated, but that could have lasting consequences if not. For example, some sexually transmitted diseases have minimal or no symptoms. If you are not tested and treated for these in a timely manner, they can result in problems later on, such as infertility issues (problems getting or staying pregnant). Sometimes, you might think the questions they ask are not relevant to your care, but information that you think is not important can often help the doctor figure out what is going on. They are basing their decisions on the information they have, and if you leave things out, they can't make their best decision. This includes answering questions for your dentist. You might think that "this doesn't have anything to do with my teeth," but things that you don't think matter do. Be truthful and know that they only ask to make sure you are safe and well cared for.

Don't leave things out, even if you think they happened too long ago or don't seem important. When the doctor asks how you have been feeling, tell them!!! Don't just say you are fine when you had a dizzy spell yesterday. They can't help you if they don't know what is going on.

> **Example:** A patient was having a CT scan of their brain and the doctor saw an area on the scan that showed damage, in an area unrelated to the condition at hand. This was very concerning to the physician because this could mean that another serious condition might need to be considered. As the doctor is questioning the patient, he asked it there were any other times that the patient had a head injury, even a long time ago. Turns out that the patient had been in a serious accident 20 years ago. The doctor asked why this was not included in the medical records. The patient said that they didn't think it mattered because it was so long ago. Learning this information meant that they did not have to consider a much more serious condition. Wow, what a relief!

Your Family's Medical History

Learning as much as you can about your family's medical history can help you obtain the best health care for yourself. There are some conditions that have a hereditary (family) component, such as cancer, diabetes, or heart disease. Now, I realize that there are many times where this information is not available and that is OK, but if you can find out, please do.

You will want to find out about your direct blood relatives' health conditions. This means your biological mother and father, grandparents,

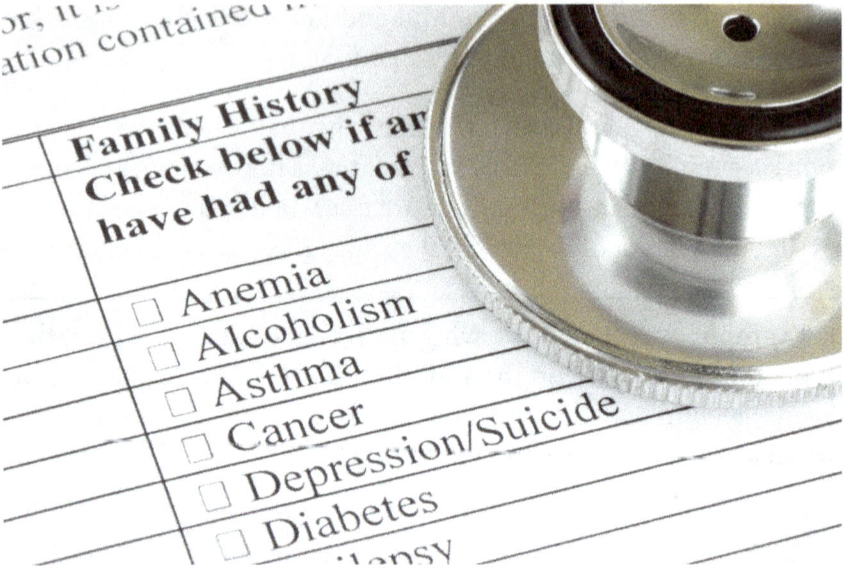

JohnKwan/Shutterstock.com

siblings (brothers and sisters) and children. If they have died, try to find out why they died. Was it old age, cancer, or a heart attack? How old were they when they passed away? All of this information can help you and your healthcare providers know what to be on the lookout for and can help prevent having some of the same problems as your family members. They may decide to do some genetic testing based on the information you provide. (Genetic testing will be discussed later in the new and emerging technologies section.)

Learn About Your Medical Conditions

Learn as much as you can about your medical conditions. If you have any chronic medical condition, such as asthma, heart disease, diabetes, or cancer, becoming knowledgeable about these conditions can help you better control and treat these conditions. This information should be found only through reputable sources. It is always best to seek the advice of your healthcare professionals on where to get the information on your specific condition.

While there is a lot of great information on internet, it is very important to remember that there is also a lot of inaccurate and/or misleading information out there too. Be careful where you find your information. For the younger generations out there, remember that influencers are not physicians and that TikTok videos are not a substitute for a doctor's visit.

Never, Never, Never, Self-Diagnose!!!

While I know it is very easy to look up your symptoms and try to find out what is going on, you really should try not to do this. Doctors and nurses spend lots of time trying to re-educate patients and explaining that they do not have some condition that they found by researching their symptoms on the internet. As tempting as it might be, just don't! Talk to your doctor about your concerns and symptoms and let them do their job. Then, they can then tell you where to find accurate, helpful information on your illness or condition.

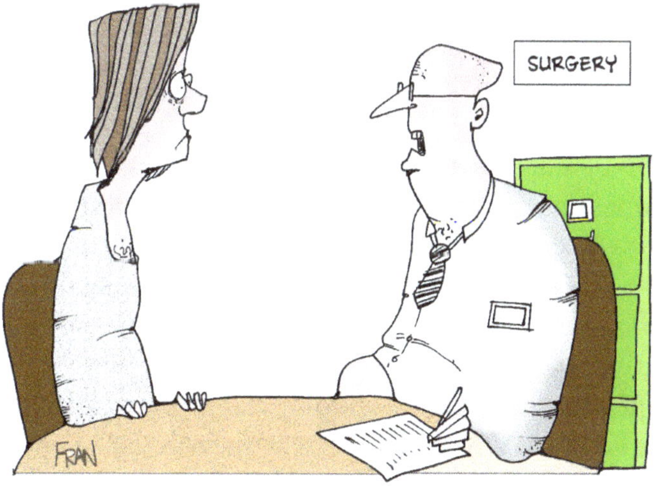

I'M GLAD YOU TOOK THE TROUBLE TO DIAGNOSE YOUR OWN SYMPTOMS USING THE INTERNET...AND YOU'D BE 100% ACCURATE...IF YOU WERE A GOAT!

Other Things You Need to Know

There are several other things that are important for you to know that can affect your health care. I will list these and tell you why they are important in this section and will show you an example of how to put this information together in a later section.

BLOOD TYPE

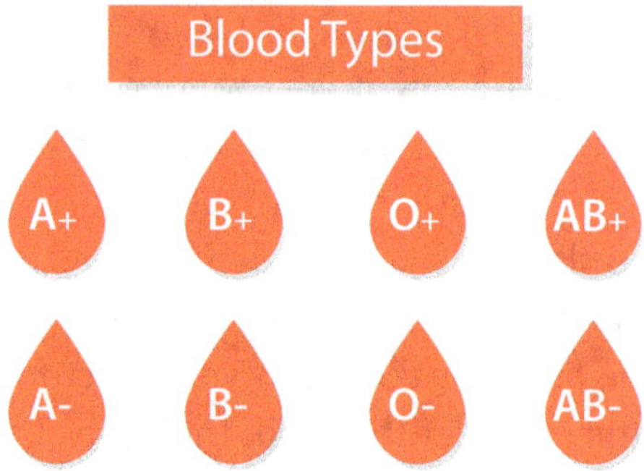

Forgetmenot29/Shutterstock.com

Do you know your own blood type? Most people don't, unless they are regular blood donors or served in the military. This information is very important to know, especially if you are having surgery. While they will always type your blood, this is something you should still be aware of so you can double check that you are receiving the correct blood type or know if you can be a donor for a friend or family member in an emergency situation.

Your blood group is determined by the presence or absence of antigens (things that can cause an immune response). The blood groups are A, B, AB, and O. Blood is also classified by the presence or absence of a protein called an Rh factor. This makes blood either negative or positive. The type of blood you have will determine what type of blood you can receive; here are a couple of examples. A person with O negative blood (O–) can only receive O negative blood, but they can donate to anyone. This is why they are called universal donors. People with AB positive (AB+) blood can receive blood of any type; this is why they are called universal recipients. Knowing your and your partner's blood type will also be important when having children. Mothers who have a negative blood type may need to have a medication to prevent problems during pregnancy if your partner has a positive blood type. Ask your obstetrician/gynecologist for more information.

MEDICATION, FOOD, AND CONTACT ALLERGIES

When most people think of allergies, they think about seasonal allergies or allergies to pets, but there are other types of allergies that are very important to your health. Medication allergies are one of these and knowing which medications you are allergic to can be vital to your health and safety. Not only do you need to know what medicine you are allergic to but you also need to know what happens if you take that medication. Do you break out in hives or have trouble breathing? I am not trying to scare you, but I do want you to know that this could be the difference between life and death.

Knowing what food allergies you have is also very important to your health care and something that your doctors should be aware of, and not just because they might need to prescribe you medicine (like an Epipen) to treat it, but because it can affect what medications you can receive. For instance, if you are allergic to eggs, you may not be able to receive certain vaccines because some vaccine are developed using eggs.

Contact allergies are something we often forget about. These are allergies to things you come in contact with, such as wool. But they also include thing like latex or adhesives. These are two things that are commonly found in a medical or dental setting, and if you are allergic, your healthcare providers may need to use latex-free gloves or use bandages with alternative adhesive material.

Example: I am very allergic to almost all antibiotics. This is not a good thing and is something that I have to really pay attention to. One time I was in a doctor's office to get an IV to help replace some nutrients, fluids, and increase my blood pressure, the nurse came in to get me hooked up to the IV and had a syringe with her. I asked her what she had and she told me that she was going to give me my antibiotics. Well, I wasn't supposed to be getting any antibiotics and, in fact, this medication was for another patient. Not only was the medication something that I am highly allergic to but it is also something, that for me, can cause severe respiratory distress. If I had not asked questions and known what I was allergic to, I might not be here to share this story with you. Scary!

SURGERIES, SIGNIFICANT MEDICAL EVENTS, MEDICAL CONDITIONS

You should also keep a record of all surgeries that you have had, when, and why you had them, along with any complications that occurred. It can let the doctors have a better idea of what to expect if you have surgery in the future or be able to determine whether issues you are having now might be related to previous surgeries. Your list of surgeries should include everything; even what you might think are minor procedures, such as a vasectomy or having your tubes tied or having your wisdom teeth removed. It should also include things that you might think are private, such as having breast implants or a breast reduction.

You should also keep a record of significant medical events. These events include broken bones, or having given birth to children, or having had a miscarriage or an abortion. You should also include having received a blood transfusion, having had kidney or gall stones or having had a concussion.

You should also keep a record of significant medical conditions. These include conditions such as high blood pressure (hypertension), low blood pressure (hypotension), diabetes, low blood sugar (hypoglycemia), heart disease, thyroid conditions (hypo or hyper thyroid), asthma, COPD (chronic obstructive pulmonary disorder), cancer, HIV, hepatitis (inflammation of the liver), clotting disorders, endometriosis, sexually transmitted diseases, or consistent painful menstruation. These are just some of the examples; there may be other conditions that I have not included here.

IMMUNIZATIONS AND VACCINES

You should also keep a record of your immunizations. This is very important not only for you but also for children and young adults who might require scheduled vaccinations. Adults will also want to have a record of vaccines that they have received and when if you know. This can include vaccines for the flu, COVID-19, pneumonia, tetanus, etc.

SOCIAL HISTORY

OK, this is not what it sounds like; it doesn't mean how many parties you attended. This is what healthcare providers label things that occur in your everyday life that affect your health and are things you and your advocates should share with your providers. Here are some examples of things to include in your social history.

Do you **smoke** or **vape**? How much? Is it two cigarettes a day or two packs a day? If you did before but have stopped, how long ago did you quit, and how much did you smoke before?

Do you drink **alcoholic** beverages? How much? Is it one drink a day, one drink a week, every once in a while? Are you a binge drinker or teetotaler?

What is you **caffeine** consumption? Do you drink 2 cups of coffee a day? What about tea, energy drinks, sodas?

Do you use **recreational drugs?** Have you ever been an IV drug user? While this information may be uncomfortable to disclose, remember that your healthcare providers must maintain your privacy, and as I mentioned in the section on medicine, this is vital for your best health care.

Do you follow strict **dietary practices**? Are you a vegan or vegetarian, keto, non-dairy, gluten-free? Are these choices or are they due to a medical condition?

Do you have **tattoos or piercing**s? This can be important because sometimes, they can introduce infections and/or result in conditions such as hepatitis. Also some ink used for tattoos have metals in them and can lead to problems if they need to perform an MRI. Also, having a hidden piercing with a metal ring or stud being ripped out during an MRI could be very painful.

Have you ever had a **blood transfusion?** They ask this because your body can develop a reaction to future blood products. They will also ask if you are having surgery if you will accept blood products. This can help the healthcare providers follow your wishes. There are some people who do not want to have a transfusion for religious or other reasons.

Again, this part might be a little uncomfortable, but it is important to be honest about your **sexual practices** as well. They may ask: Do you have multiple partners? Do you have a sexually transmitted disease? Do you regularly use protection? Do you have anal sex? Could you be pregnant?

Have you **traveled** outside the United States? Again, this is not to be nosey but to help determine if you could have been exposed to diseases or parasites that are not normally found in the United States.

They may also ask your **living situation**. Again, you might think that this is none of their business, but it can affect your health. It will help them determine whether you have help when recovering from a procedure or might be at risk for domestic violence or for some emotional struggles. Again, I encourage you to be honest because your privacy will be protected and they are just trying to provide you with the best care.

2

Health Care in the Age of Technology

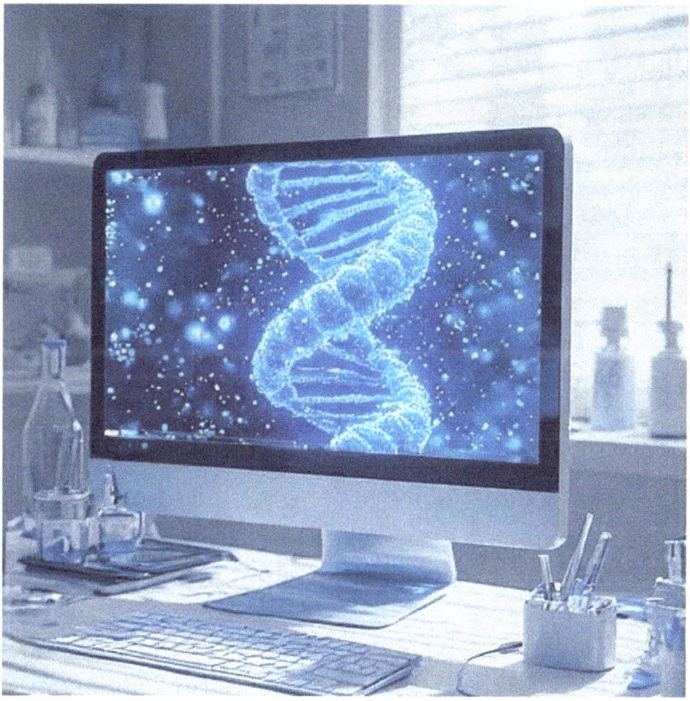

Medical Information

Medical care is largely based on the collection and processing of information in order to provide the best treatment. This information can come in the form of vital signs (such as temperature, blood pressure, and heart rate), the results of tests (such as blood work or urinalysis), and observation of the patient (seeing that the throat and nose are red and inflamed). It also includes understanding the medications and supplements a patient is taking and what allergies they have to medications and foods, etc. A lot of this information is also provided by the patients themselves through conversations and by answering what may seem like an endless list of questions. This information is then put together into your medical records.

The age of technology has brought many exciting changes to health care, one of those being electronic medical records. This new way of keeping track of your medical information can be great. It can allow healthcare providers to reduce the paperwork (often, you will be asked to fill out your questionnaires on an iPad or computer), review your medical history quickly, and send prescriptions to the pharmacy faster. It does, however, come with its own challenges.

The fact that many patients do not have access to computers or "smart" phones means that they may have to plan to spend additional time at the doctor's office filling out this "paperwork." There are also many different systems that can house these electronic medical records, not all of which are compatible. In other words, the different systems may be unable to communicate with each other. This can mean that one doctor's office may be unable to see what you have provided to the other doctor's office and hence that you may have to fill out the same information multiple times.

You might ask why it is a big deal if these systems can't talk to each other. Well, here are some things for you to think about. Sometimes, these things are just an inconvenience and mean that you have to fill out more paperwork. But in some cases, it can result in a delay in care, especially if you are having to be referred from one doctor to another. It can also lead to more serious issues, such as the prescribing of medications that may have interactions or being prescribed multiple medications that treat the same condition leading to problems resulting from too much medication. While this is often caught at the pharmacy level, it may not be if you are using multiple pharmacies. The use of multiple pharmacies can happen when you are shopping for the best price on medications.

Problems can also arise in your doctor's office even if you have already filled out all the paperwork. What if their system goes down or the internet goes out (some systems are dependent on the internet to access your records)? This can mean that they have no access to some of this critical information that you have provided, such as what medications you are taking or what you are allergic to. This means that you have to be ready to provide this information at a moment's notice. Do you remember all the names and doses of the medicine you are taking and why?

This is why I suggest that you put together your own set of medical records that you can take along each time you visit the doctors. I will discuss a little later on all the information you should include in your medical records and have provided an example of how to set them up in the back of this book.

While I am somewhat "old school" and prefer paper versions (I keep mine in a notebook that I can add pages to as I get new information, such as new bloodwork results.), I realize the younger generations may be more comfortable with electronic versions, such as apps on your phone. Just remember that you may be faced with some of the same trouble at the doctor's offices; this information can become inaccessible if the battery on your phone dies or your phone is damaged. However, if you choose this method, there are a variety of health apps available for your phones. Just be careful and make sure that the information is secure, protected, inaccessible to anyone at large.

Telemedicine

Telemedicine is another one of the advances that technology has brought to health care. In the most simple terms, it is the ability to see and treat patients at distances using the phone and videoconferencing capabilities. This technology has given rural communities the access to health care where medical services are not readily available. It has also provided more rapid access to health care by making it easier for patients to get appointments.

However, it also comes with its own challenges. As I mentioned earlier, medical care is largely based on the collection and processing of information in order to provide the best treatment. One of the challenges with telemedicine is that the remote care can limit the amount of information the healthcare providers can obtain. They cannot take your blood pressure, listen to your heart or breathing, take your temperature, or draw blood or obtain a urine sample for laboratory testing. This makes getting the best care more of a challenge.

If you choose to use these telemedicine services on a regular basis, you might want to invest in a few reasonably cost-effective devices that can help your doctor help you.

The most simple of these devices is a **digital thermometer**, which can allow your provider to determine if you have a fever. A **digital scale** is a simple tool to help monitor your weight. Even the inexpensive models are easy to read and can be very accurate. Another is an **automated blood pressure monitor** that can provide your blood pressure and heart rate. There are a number of accurate monitors on the market, and any device you purchase can be verified to be accurate by your healthcare provider.

If you have lung problems such as asthma or COPD (chronic obstructive pulmonary disorder), another helpful device is a **pulse oximeter (PulseOx)**. This a small device that fits on your finger and can determine the amount of oxygen in your blood.

If you have problems with your blood sugar, whether low—hypoglycemia—or high—hyperglycemia or diabetes—a **blood glucose (blood sugar) monitor** could be a lifesaver. There are also more high-tech versions that will be mentioned in the new technology section.

There are also some more expensive devices on the market that might be useful in some circumstances. One of these devices is a **smart watch**. Many versions have apps that can track you heart rate over time and record you exercise sessions, and some can also run a single lead ECG (**electrocardiogram, often called an EKG**). There are other devices that can connect to your phone to provide this information as well. However, I must caution that these are never a substitute for medical ECGs that are performed by your healthcare provider.

There are even **tiny cameras** that connect to your phone that can allow the doctor to see you ears, nose, and throat.

New and Emerging Technologies

There are always new and emerging technologies becoming available in health care. Examples of these are robot-assisted surgery, wearable technologies, and genetic testing. While we may sometimes be slow to develop a comfort level with all the changes, embracing some of the these new technologies can be extremely beneficial and can empower us to receive the best care possible.

ROBOTICS

Robot-assisted surgery does not take the place of the surgeon but allows the surgeon to use less invasive techniques that can improve recovery time. This may not always be available, depending on your individual circumstances, but it never hurts to ask your doctor if this is an option.

WEARABLE TECHNOLOGY

There are smart watches that monitor you heart rate and exercise and even some that can run a single-lead ECG. There are also wearable devices that monitor blood glucose levels and can help your doctor collect information to improve your health care. There are so many options that may benefit you in achieving your healthcare goals. Be sure to talk to your healthcare provider about these wearables and how they may be useful in your health care journey.

GENETIC TESTING

Another one of these advances is genetic testing. Now I am not talking about the novel tests that look at your ancestry; I am talking about the medical genetic tests. The field of genetic testing has improved greatly over the last few years. With the improvements come the potential to improve and personalize your health care based on your own genetic makeup. Tests are now available to determine how medicines work with your genetics, called PGX or pharmacogenomics. There are also genetic panels that can help determine your cardiovascular risks, as well as your risk of developing some types of cancer or risk of developing other diseases.

You should talk to your healthcare provider to determine if some of these new technologies are available to help you improve your health and achieve your healthcare goals.

3

Patient Advocates

What Is an Advocate and Why You Should Have One

What is a patient advocate? A patient advocate is someone who can be there with you when you go to the doctor or hospital. This doesn't have to be someone who is a trained medical professional. It can also be a trusted friend or family member. They are there to help make sure you are receiving the appropriate and best care, to "advocate" for you.

Having an advocate for children and the disabled is a must. However, we might forget that teenagers, young adults, and the elderly also need advocates. Even us "regular ole adults" can benefit from having an advocate go with them to any health care appointment.

You actually might find it very helpful to have an advocate go with you, especially in certain circumstances, such as when you might be receiving some stressful news or are having surgery. Some people are just nervous going to the doctor and having a trusted person go with you can ease your mind.

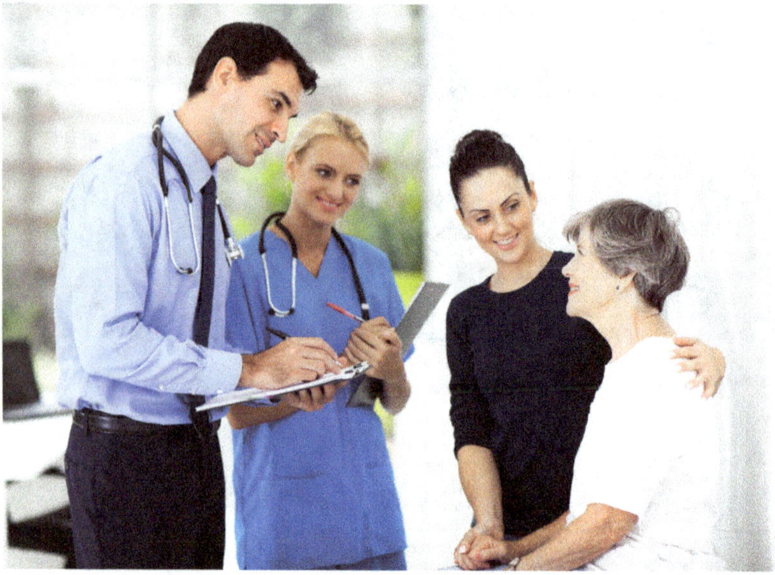

michaeljung/Shutterstock.com

Advocates can do things as simple as hold your hand, provided support, help you ask questions, or listen to the doctor as they are explaining things. A second set of eyes and ears are always helpful. They may catch things that you miss or think of questions that you may have overlooked.

They can also be there during more serious situations. Maybe you have to have surgery and will be in the hospital for a period of time. They can help you when you are coming out of anesthesia or taking medicines that make you feel groggy or any situation that may make it harder to understand what is happening. They can help you if you need to get up and go to the restroom, get you a drink of water, or call the nurse if something is wrong. They can help communicate your wishes when you can't. They can be a great safety net too. They can make sure you are getting the correct medication or, in the case of someone allergic to medication, that you are not getting the wrong medication.

The age of COVID-19 and lockdowns really heightened my awareness of how much advocates are needed. No patient should be isolated and asked to make critical decisions about their care without having an advocate present. They should not be dropped off at the hospital door for an emergency or surgery and not allowed to have an advocate with them. **Remember that patients do have rights!!! And the ability to have an advocate with you is one of them!!!**

> While I have many stories about how having an advocate with you can make the difference in obtaining the best and most appropriate health care, I will share one example when having an advocate with me made all the difference to my safety. I was hospitalized with very serious complications following the birth of my son. I was in very bad shape, heavily medicated, and a bit out of it, so I wasn't able to be as active in my own health care as I would normally be. The nurse came in and started to give me some medication in my IV. I was way too groggy to ask her what she was giving me. Well, it turns out that it was medication for another patient and something that I am deathly allergic to. If it had not been for my friend/advocate, who checked the medicine bag and disconnected my IV, I might not be here to tell you this story. My advocate also had to make sure that this critical mistake was not covered up and brought this to the attention of the hospital administrators. This allowed for the retraining of the nursing staff and the implementation of additional safety procedures to ensure this type of mistake would not be made again. I cannot express how grateful I am that my advocate was with me that day!

What if I am an Advocate?

If you are serving as someone's advocate, there are a few things that you should do to make sure that the person you are advocating for is getting the best care.

Know their medicines, allergies, surgeries, significant medical events, etc. All the things mentioned above that you would want to know about your own health. I always bring a notepad with me so I can write down information and can go over it with the person I am advocating for or their family members.

You may want to help them put together a medical record similar to the example I will be giving in the next section. I would also suggest you keep a copy at their home, with them, and one with you, just in case an emergency happens that denies you access to the one at their home.

If you are serving as an advocate during the patient's hospital stay, be sure to ask about any medications being given. The staff should always check the patient's name and allergy wrist bands, confirm the patient's name and date of birth, and verify what medication is being given and why before administering any medication. If they fail to do any of these safety checks, be sure to speak up. Remember you are the last line of defense!

Advocates as a Service

One of the advances that has emerged in recent years is professional advocates. These are often medical professionals or persons that have been trained to help you navigate the healthcare system, understand your options or conditions, and make informed decisions. They may be employed by an insurance company, hospital, or treatment center such as a dialysis center to help patients.

There are also advocates that can be hired by individuals similar to health aids, to assist with taking patients to doctors' appointments, helping with medication organization, and giving updates to family members. These services may be an option if the patient lives some distance from family or friends that would normally be an advocate. As with any person that you entrust with aiding a family member (babysitter, nanny, etc.), be sure to check them out thoroughly, verify licenses, and check out references.

These advocates can be a great asset, but they are not a substitute for having your own friend or family member with you.

4

Preparing for Your Doctor's Visits

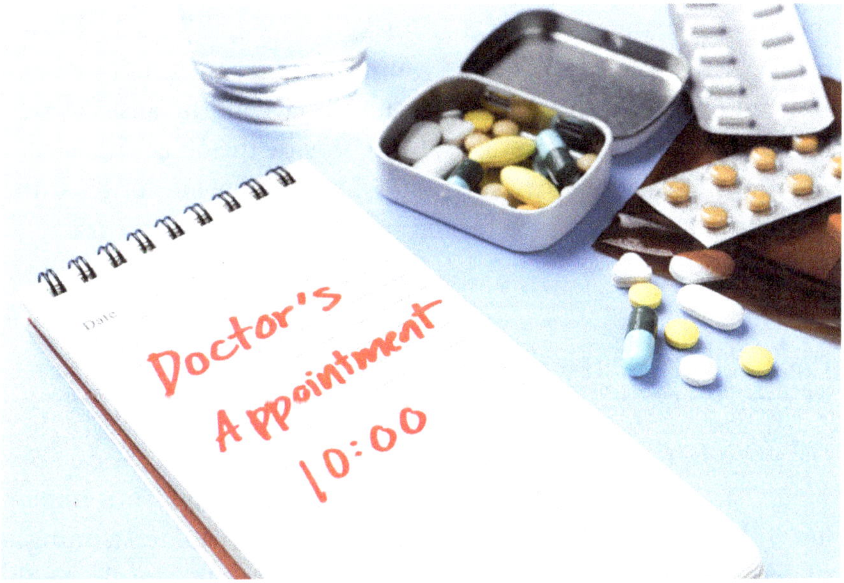

everycayplus/Shutterstock.com

Must Haves for Every Visit

There are a few things that you should bring with you to every doctor's visit. These include your driver's license or government issued ID (identification card); your insurance cards (primary and secondary if you have them); your list of medications with dosages, instructions, and why you take them; list of allergies to medications, foods, etc., form of payment (even if you have insurance, most visits will require some type of payment for your copay); list of questions that you want to ask; and a notepad. I like having a notepad so I can write down important information that might be shared or new medications with instructions and jot down my next appointment time.

You will also need to plan on going a few minutes early to fill out paperwork, especially if this is the first time you will be seeing a healthcare provider. Some offices will ask you to fill out this information online before your visit. I know that it can be hard to remember all of the answers to the questions that are being asked; this is why I like to bring my medical records that I put together for myself. It saves me time filling out the paperwork because I have all the answers right in front of me. And often times, I will provide the office with a copy. This can be very handy, especially when you have a long list that doesn't fit in the tiny space for the answer on their paperwork.

Pack Your Patience

We all know that your time is valuable and so is your healthcare providers'. In order for us to obtain the best care possible, it is important to be a "patient patient." In other words, be understanding of the time it takes to provide the best care. If we want our doctors to be able to spend time with us, to listen to our concerns, answer our questions, and give you undivided attention, we have to allow them to do this with their other patients as well. We also have to understand that in emergencies, there may be delays or a need to reschedule appointments. This is especially true for certain types of doctors such as surgeons, cardiologists, and obstetricians. While I know it can be inconvenient, please be understanding and kind not only to the providers but to their staff as well. Doing so will make everyone's day better and will improve the care you receive.

Develop a Habit of Asking About Medications You Are Receiving

You should develop the habit of asking questions any time you're given a medication. If it is a prescription that they are going to send to your pharmacy, ask why you are being given this medicine and ask that the doctor explain how you should take this medicine, including whether it should be taken at a certain time of day, with or without food. You should also verify that this will not interact with any of the medicines you are taking (having your medication list is important) and remind them of you allergies. This will ensure that you are not being given a medication related to something you are allergic to and could prevent a reaction.

If you are being given a medication in the doctor's office or hospital, you should always take additional precautions. This is especially critical if the medication is being given as a shot or in an IV (intravenously) because these medications are usually faster acting. Ask the person giving you the medication to confirm that the medication is intended for you. They should always ask you for your name and birth date and if you are wearing a wrist band, they should look at it as well. This is a safety measure to ensure you are getting the correct medication. If they forget, ask them again to verify this medication is for you. You don't want to have an experience like the one I shared earlier. Ask why you are being given this medication, whether you will be receiving another dose, and if so, when.

I understand that you might think they know who you are and should know what you are taking, but it never hurts to be safe.

5

Preparing for Surgeries and Hospital Stays

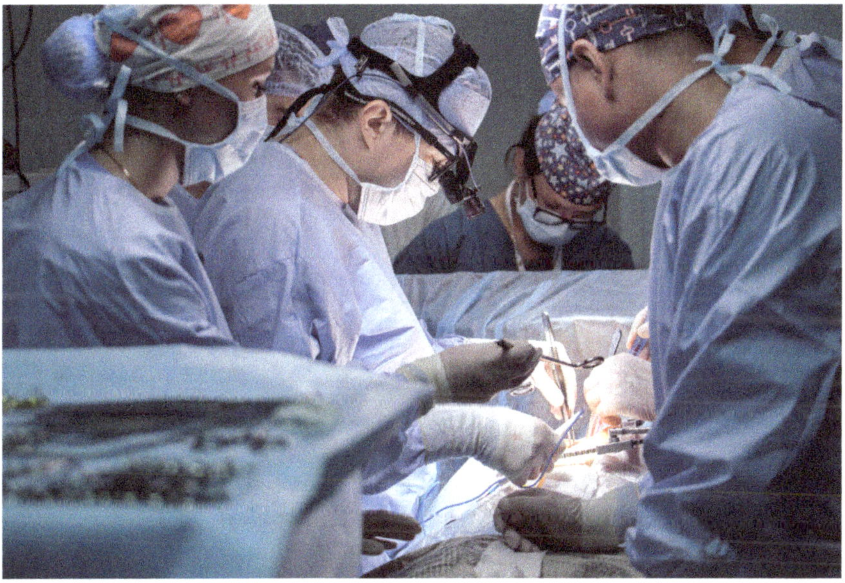

Biland/Shutterstock.com

You should have the same information you would have with you for a regular office visit. There are also a few additional things that can be helpful to have or to do as you prepare for surgery.

During you preop visit they will collect all the information they need to prepare for your surgery. Yep! This means more paperwork. Depending on the type of surgery, they may draw blood and do some other things like taking x-rays and an ECG. They will also give you detailed directions on what to do to prepare for your surgery, such as when to stop eating or drinking, ask you to bath with a special cleanser, and tell you what medicines to take or what medicines to stop taking. Be sure to follow these directions very carefully! They are very important for your safety and if not followed, may mean that your surgery will be delayed. Some medications that need to be stopped before surgery are blood thinners and weight loss medications.

Even if you are not scheduled to stay overnight, you should still pack a small bag with the following items. Your advocate will be able to keep the bag with them while you are undergoing your procedure.

A case for your glasses or contacts, if you wear them, should be included in your bag. They will need to be removed before surgery. Also bring a case for dentures, removable teeth, or bridges. You will need to remove these for surgery, and you don't want to get them accidentally thrown away in a paper towel or tissue.

You also need a comfortable change of clothes with socks and underwear. It is always better to have them and not need them than to need them and not have them.

I always like to have a notepad and pen with me so my advocate can take notes or jot down names of care providers I want to remember or for any other notes I might want to make. I recently had an unplanned extended hospital stay and my notepad and pen came in very handy when I needed to make a list of things my husband needed to take care of while I was out of commission and for the extra things I needed for him to gather up and bring to me for my longer stay.

If you are going to have a cell phone with you, you will also want to pack a charger. I personally like to have an extra battery bank so I can charge my device without having to plug into an outlet. When you are in a hospital bed or on a stretcher in an exam room, the plugs are rarely within reach.

If you know that you will be a guest at the hospital for a few days, you will want to pack a few self-care items, such as toothbrush and travel size toothpaste, deodorant, hairbrush, etc. If allowed, you may also want your own PJs; hospital gowns aren't always the most comfortable and can be very revealing.

The Part Nobody Wants to Talk About

OK, here is where I am going to talk about the part nobody wants to talk about, and this used to include me. When preparing for surgery and hospital stays, we should all prepare for the worst case scenario. No, nobody wants to think about what might go wrong, but we still have to; in fact your healthcare providers are obligated to explain to you all the risks of whatever procedure you are about to undergo. This means that you not only need to understand the risks but that you should also address what you want to happen if things don't go as planned.

While a lot of us think that "it can't happen to me," the reality is that sometimes it does. We should be thinking, "I don't want my family having to make life altering decisions in the middle of a stressful situation." Often, this is an urgent decision that has to be made in a very short time frame. But, we can take care of some of these decisions upfront and not put them through that stress of not knowing how you would want things handled.

You see, I have had more experience with Murphy's Law (you know, if it can go wrong, it will go wrong) than most. I have been the one having things go wrong and the family member having to make decisions for others when things don't go as planned for them. In the callout box, I will share a very personal story about one of such times that I think will really help you see why this is so important.

I hope that this little personal story shows you just how important it is that you communicate your wishes not only to the healthcare provider but also to your advocates and family members that have a vested interest in your well-being.

This doesn't mean you have to plan all of your end-of-life choices before you have any surgery, but you do want to think about who will be making medical decisions for you if you are not capable of making your own. Think about things like whether you are OK receiving blood transfusions or about what measures you want taken if things do not go as planned. Do some research on living wills, advanced directives, and do not resuscitate orders (DNRs). Many hospitals have good resources and will ask if you want more information. I encourage you to take them up on their offer. Being informed is powerful and can help you consider things you may not have thought of before.

OK, you will need to understand some background to get the full impact of the story. Not all that long ago, I had torn my rotator cuff and had planned to have it fixed and had already scheduled the surgery, but my body had other plans. I ended up having a very large uterine fibroid that caused me to lose a great deal of blood. Well, the shoulder surgery had to be put on the back burner while we addressed this urgent situation, so we scheduled the hysterectomy. My doctor was optimistic that we could use the robotic surgery (one of those technologies that I spoke about) and I should be good to go right away, but Murphy's Law was hard at work. Through no fault of my doctor's, things went sideways very quickly and the trauma surgeon was called. I will leave out all the gory details, but long story short, four surgeries, six hospitalizations, and more than eight months later, I was finally back in one piece.

Now I know that sounds like the worst case scenario, but there is more to the story. Here is the really important part I want to share about preparing for the part nobody wants to talk about. During this challenging medical journey, there was a brief period of time when I got to "Meet my Maker—My Lord and Savior," hold my Daddy's hand one more time, and come back. As this was about to happen, I was trying very hard to explain to my husband how bad things really were and he was truly not prepared to hear it; he just wanted me to be OK. I knew in that moment that we should have had that hard conversation long before this happened. But you see, by the grace of God, I got to have another chance, and I have been able to share my wishes with my family and been called on to share this book with you, so you and your family can be prepared as well. And all that time that I spent recovering? Well it also gave me time to get to work on this book (that had been around in the back of my mind for so long) so I could share it with you.

And one last thing—I want to make sure you understand you have the power to choose as much or as little care for lifesaving measures as you are comfortable with. It is not an all or nothing decision. In fact, my husband and son are empowered to try everything they need to try, but to know I am OK being let go. I wanted to make sure they have the opportunity to try if they need to, because I know that is important to them, but I'm good; because at the end of the day I know where I am headed and who is waiting for me.

OK, that is enough of the hard stuff. Now let's talk about next steps.

6

Putting Together Your Own Medical Record

Let's Get Started

While I do understand that the thought of putting together your own health record can sound overwhelming, just remember that it doesn't have to be done all at once and that you can start with the basics and add on as you go.

As I mentioned earlier, I like having a paper version so it can be accessed at any time, but you can always use any number of health apps that are available. Let's start with the things you must have for every appointment

Identifying Information

Start with your identifying information. I am talking about your name, birthday, social security number, driver's license or ID, and your insurance cards. Be sure to include the back of the cards; this is where contact phone numbers and websites are located. I also like to include a current picture.

The rest of the information can be put all in the order that you find most convenient for you, but I will share the order that I use.

Emergency Contacts

I like to put my emergency contact information right up front. This includes their name, their relationship to me, and their contact information. I also note who is the primary point of contact for appointment and preop scheduling if I am not available.

Medical History

Blood Type: As I mentioned before, many people do not know their blood type, but if you do, put it in you record. If you don't, put a placeholder for it so you can ask your doctor to let you know or they can order it in your next blood workup.

Allergies: I like to put this information close to the beginning and written in red to call attention to it. Include a section for allergies to medication as well as a section for food and contact allergies.

Current/Relevant Medical Information: This section would include a list of chronic conditions such as diabetes, hypertension, COPD, cancer, etc. List all of these that you are aware of and when they began if you know. I also note how they are managed, such as hypertension, well controlled with current medication.

List of Medications: Next make a list of all your medications, names, strength, dosing information, etc. This includes any herbal supplements, vitamins, hormones, and recreational drugs; all the items I mentioned earlier.

Surgeries: List each of your surgeries and dates. If you do not know that exact date, at least try to give the year they occurred. This list would include C-sections if you had them. If you know of any complications, you can add those in as well. For instance, you might list that the anesthesiologist noted that you were difficult to intubate due to enlarged tonsils.

Major Hospitalizations and Injuries: This section will include anytime you were injured in a car accident, had a concussion, or broken bones. It can also include anytime you delivered children if not by C-section, infections, etc. Be sure to include dates if you can remember them. This is where you would include information about miscarriages as well.

Social History: This section would be where you list whether you drink alcohol, or smoke, or your caffeine intake, tattoos, piercings, recreational drug use, etc. As I mentioned before, while you might not be completely comfortable sharing this information, it is still very important and can really make a difference in receiving the appropriate care.

Family History: This is where you include any known family history. If a family member has passed away, include the cause of death if known and their age.

List of Physicians/Healthcare Providers

It is always good to have a list of all your health care providers and their contact information. This is vitally important when considering continuity of care. In other words, this way, all of your doctors can communicate if they need to speak provider to provider. You should also list your dentist, chiropractor, and alternative health providers here as well.

Pharmacy

It is also important to include the information on the pharmacy that you use regularly as well as the contact information for the pharmacy. This will help ensure that any prescriptions are sent to the correct location.

Example Medical Record

On the next few pages, you will see an example of a medical record that can be put together. This is a basic one that could be kept in a notebook, with completely fictional information. You can create your own to fit your information and needs.

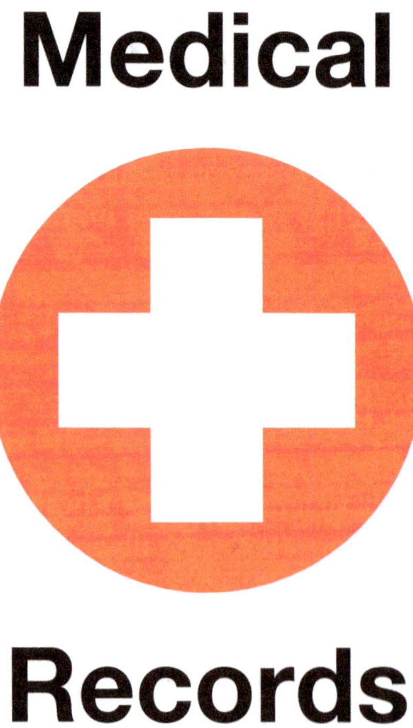

Jane Doe

DOB: July 4, 1950

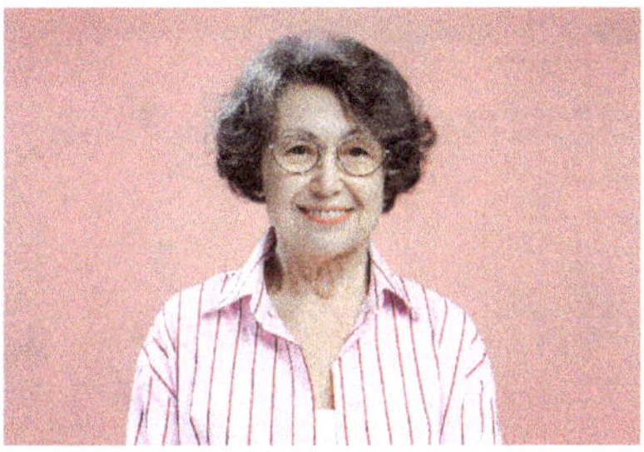

AYO Production/Shutterstock.com

Address: 1234 Best Street
Anywhere, Texas 90210

Phone: (555) 555-5555

Cell Phone: (444) 444-4444

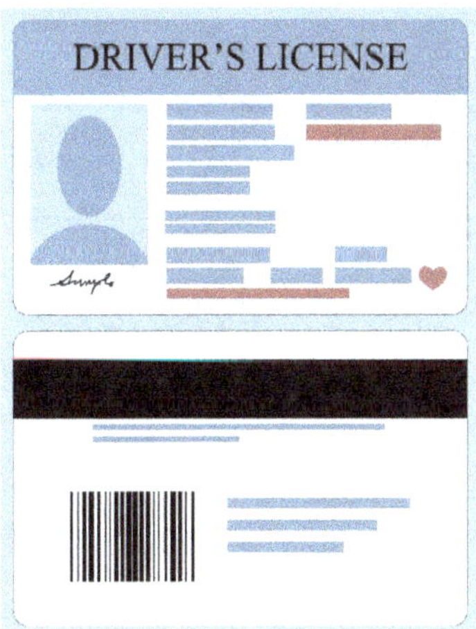

Becris/Shutterstock.com

Email: JaneDoe@email.com

Sex: Female

Height: 5'02"

Weight: ~150 lbs

Eyes: Blue

Date of Birth: July 4, 1950

Race/Ethnicity: White/Not Hispanic

DL: TX 12345678

SS#: 123-45-6789

Married: Husband - John Doe

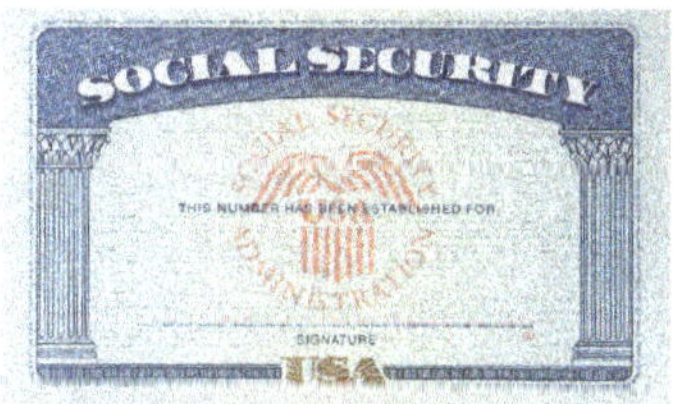

Artiom Photo/Shutterstock.com

Emergency Contacts

John Doe - husband (222) 222-2222

James Doe- son (333) 333-3333

Jane Doe

DOB: July 4, 1950

Insurance Information

Primary Insurance

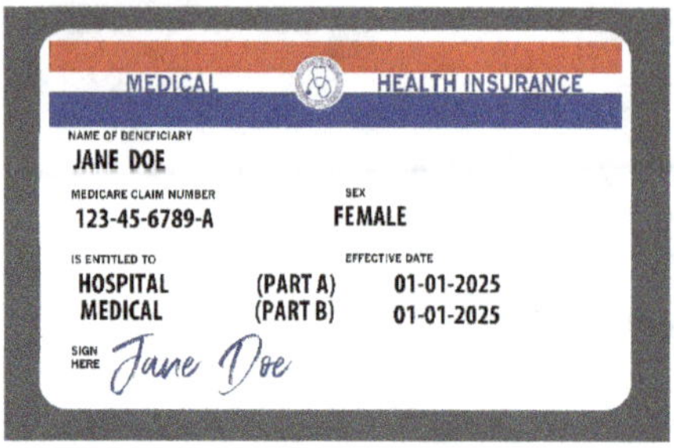

robertindiana/Shutterstock.com

Secondary Insurance

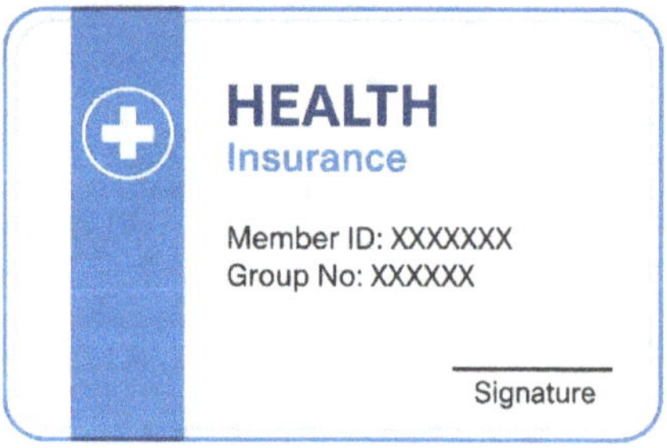

lukyfebrie22/Shutterstock.com

Prescription Card

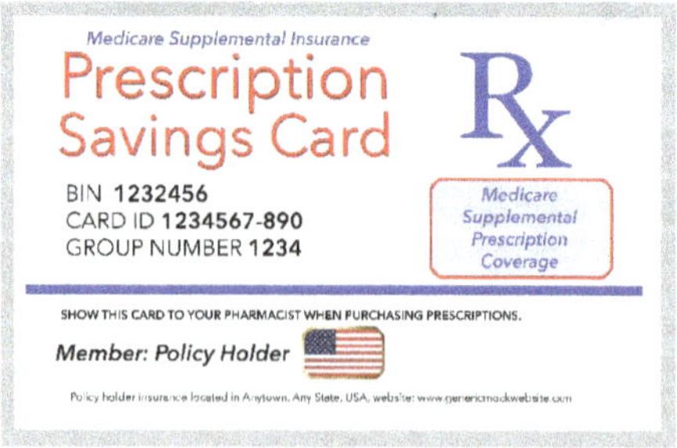

robertindiana/Shutterstock.com

Jane Doe

DOB: July 4, 1950

Medical History

Blood Type: A+

Allergies:

Tetanus - had reaction when she was given tetanus as a child and has never had any other vaccines or boosters since

Neosporin/Cyclosporin/Polysporin - causes severe reaction, including rash, hives, systemic swelling, tongue swelling

Current Relevant Medical Information:

Insomnia: well controlled with medication

Hypertension: well controlled with medication

Current Medications:

aspirin - 81 mg tablet - 1 tablet by mouth daily

losartan - 100mg tablet - 1 tablet by mouth daily (for hypertension) (Cozarr)

zolpidem - 5mg at bedtime for sleep

multivitamin - 2 tablets a day

Surgeries and Hospitalizations:

5/7/1990 **Back surgery** for L4/L5 disc herniation

1/1/1970 - C-section - delivered a healthy son

2/16/ 1972 - car accident - resulting in a concussion

Jane Doe

DOB: July 4, 1950

Social History:

Smoker: previously a heavy smoker (from 1977- 2000), has not smoked since 2000

Alcohol: currently a social drinker (varies from 1 to 3 drinks a month

Caffeine: 2 cups of coffee per day and drinks cokes and tea

Drug Use: used recreational drugs in the past ~ early 1970's

Tattoos and Piercings: none

Travel: has NOT recently traveled outside the United States

Family History:

Father: Deceased 1927- 1971 cause of death - heart attack

Mother: Deceased 1921 - 2003 cause of death - old age and dementia

Physicians

Primary Care:

Richard Thomas, MD
403 Main St.
Anywhere, TX 90210
(555) 867-5309

Cardiologist:

Karen Kim, MD
605 E 2nd St.
Anywhere, TX 90211
(555) 222-7777

Pharmacy

Hometown Pharmacy
500 Main St.
Anywhere, TX 90211
(555) 333-111

Conclusion

I hope you find the information I have provided in this guide book helpful. I am blessed to have had the opportunity to share it with you and sincerely hope it empowers you to "Help your Doctor Help You!"

How to Spread the Word

If you found the information in this book helpful, there are several ways you can help share the message. It can be as simple as gifting a book to a friend or family member, sharing the book with your care providers or pharmacists, or you may consider sharing in a larger way, maybe with your church, senior center, or other organizations.

Care providers, pharmacies, healthcare systems, local stores, ect. can reach out to Innovative Ink for bulk purchase information.

Dr. Johnson can also do speaking events for organizations, churches, community outreach (health fairs), book signings and the like. If you would like to discuss this option, please reach out to Dr. Johnson directly:

DustieJohnson@aol.com
P.O. Box 52213
Midland, Texas 78710
(432) 967-1618

About the Author

Dr. Dustie Johnson was born and raised in Midland, Texas, where she still resides. She has both a masters and a doctorate in Reproductive Physiology and is an applied scientist at heart. Her research has a led to a US patent as well as several international patents. She has presented at many national and international conferences and has authored a number of publications in well-respected scientific journals. Dr. Johnson has a very strong medical and scientific background, which included teaching Anatomy and Physiology, Reproductive Physiology, and Animal Science as well as serving as Medical/Science Liaison and Consultant in pharmaceutical, medical device, and business world for nearly 30 years.

Dustie has had the amazing privilege of being a long-time patient advocate for family and friends and has been a patient more than a few times herself. This, along with her unique work experience, has afforded her the opportunity to gather a great deal of knowledge and information. She has a passion for sharing this knowledge and she believes in the philosophy "what good is knowledge if it is not shared." The calling to share this knowledge is what led her to write the book that you have just read.

www.ingramcontent.com/pod-product-compliance
Lightning Source LLC
LaVergne TN
LVHW022323200926
848481LV00004B/1409